My Slow Cooker Diet Cookbook

Don't Miss These Quick and Easy Recipes to Make Incredible Slow Cooker Appetizers

Sean Miller

Table of Contents

Banana and Coconut Milk Steel-Cut Oats

Preparation time:

15 minutes

Cooking time:

3 hours

Servings:

4 people

Ingredients:

- 2 medium ripe bananas, sliced
- 2 cans coconut milk, unsweetened
- 1 cup steel-cut oats
- 2 tablespoons brown sugar
- ½ teaspoon cinnamon

Directions:

1. Place all ingredients in the slow cooker.
2. Add a dash of salt if needed.
3. Give a good stir.
4. Cook on low within 3 hours.
5. Once cooked, serve with a tablespoon of melted butter.

Nutrition:

- Calories:101
- Carbs: 15.3 g
- Protein: 2.6 g
- Fat: 5.9 g

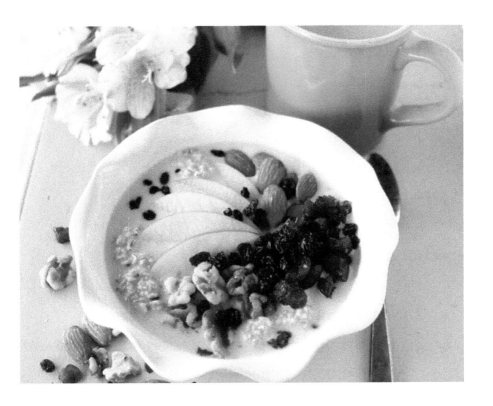

Spinach and Mozzarella Frittata

Preparation time:

10 minutes

Cooking time:

4 hours

Servings:

4 people

Ingredients:

- 6 eggs, beaten
- 2 tablespoons milk
- 1 cup baby spinach
- 1 cup mozzarella cheese
- 1 Roma tomatoes, diced

Directions:

1. Mix the eggs and milk in a mixing bowl.
2. Season with salt and pepper to taste.
3. Put the egg batter into the slow cooker and add the baby spinach, cheese, and tomatoes.
4. Cook on low within 4 hours.

Nutrition:

- Calories: 139
- Carbs: 4 g
- Protein: 12 g
- Fat: 8 g

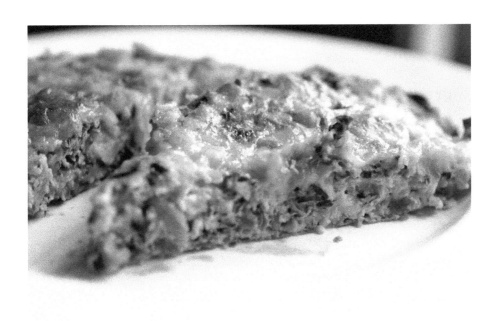

Quinoa Energy Bars

Preparation time:

15 minutes

Cooking time:

8 hours

Servings:

4 people

Ingredients:

- 2 cups quinoa flakes, rinsed
- ½ cup nuts of your choice
- ½ cup dried fruits of your choice
- ¼ cup butter, melted
- 1/3 cup maple syrup

Directions:

1. In a mixing bowl, combine all ingredients.
2. Compress the fixing in a parchment-lined slow cooker.
3. Cook on low within 8 hours.

Nutrition:

- Calories: 306
- Carbs: 39.9 g
- Protein: 7.3 g
- Fat: 13.9 g

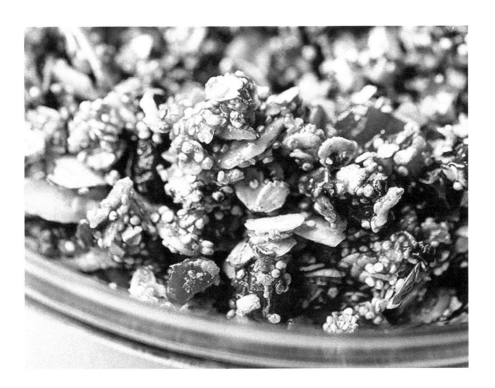

Overnight Apple Oatmeal

Preparation time:

15 minutes

Cooking time:

8 hours

Servings:

4 people

Ingredients:

- 4 apples, peeled and diced
- ¾ cup brown sugar
- 2 cups old-fashioned oats
- 4 cups evaporated milk
- 1 tablespoon cinnamon

Directions:

1. Stir in all fixing in the slow cooker.
2. Cook on low within 8 hours.
3. Add in butter if desired.

Nutrition:

- Calories: 521
- Carbs: 109.5 g

- Protein: 16.4 g
- Fat: 11.6 g

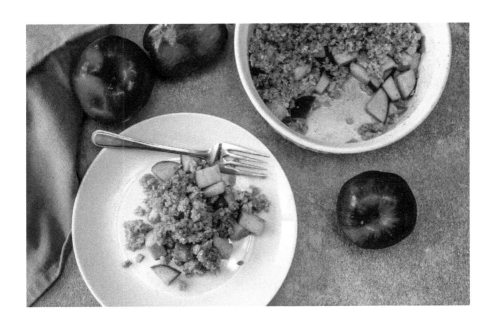

Apple Walnut Strata

Preparation time:

15 minutes

Cooking time:

2 hours

Servings:

4 people

Ingredients:

- ¼ cup light cream
- ¼ cup of orange juice
- 3 eggs, beaten
- 3 tablespoons sugar
- ½ teaspoon cinnamon
- 1 teaspoon vanilla
- 4 cups cubed French bread
- 1 cup granola
- ½ cup chopped toasted walnuts
- 2 Granny Smith apples, peeled and cubed

Directions:

1. Oiled 3 or 4-quart slow cooker using a nonstick cooking spray.

2. In a medium bowl, combine cream, orange juice, eggs, sugar, cinnamon, and vanilla and blend well with a whisk.
3. Set aside.
4. Place the bread in the prepared slow cooker's bottom and sprinkle it with the granola, walnuts, and apples—repeat layers.
5. Pour egg mixture overall.
6. Cover and cook on high within 1½ to 2 hours or until just set.
7. Serve.

Nutrition:

- Calories: 357.67
- Fat: 16.56 g
- Protein: 11.97 g
- Carbs: 0 g

Nutty Oatmeal

Preparation time:

15 minutes

Cooking time:

9 hours & 9 minutes

Servings:

4 people

Slow cooker size: 3 1/2-quart

Ingredients:

- 1½ cups steel-cut oatmeal
- 2 tablespoons butter
- 1 cup chopped walnuts
- 6 cups of water
- ½ cup brown sugar
- 1 teaspoon salt
- 1 teaspoon cinnamon
- 1 teaspoon nutmeg

Directions:

1. Put the oatmeal in a large skillet over medium-high heat.

2. Toast, continually stirring, for 8–9 minutes or until oatmeal is fragrant and begins to brown around the edges.
3. Remove to 3½-quart slow cooker.
4. Dissolve butter and add chopped walnuts in the same pan.
5. Toast over medium heat, continually stirring, until nuts are toasted.
6. Combine with all remaining ingredients except spices in 3– the 4-quart slow cooker. Cover and cook on low for 7–9 hours, until oatmeal is tender.
7. Stir in spices, cover, and let stand for 10 minutes.
8. Serve topped with a bit of butter, maple syrup, brown sugar, and more chopped nuts.

Nutrition:

- Calories: 388
- Carbs: 32 g
- Fat: 26 g
- Protein: 13 g

Bacon and Waffle Strata

Preparation time:

15 minutes

Cooking time:

5 hours

Servings:

4 people

Ingredients:

- 4 slices bacon
- 5 frozen waffles, toasted
- 1 cup shredded Colby cheese
- ¼ cup chopped green onions
- 1 (5-ounce) can evaporate milk
- ½ package cream cheese softened
- 4 eggs
- ½ teaspoon dry mustard

Directions:

1. Cook bacon until crisp in your large skillet.
2. Drain on paper towels, crumble, and set aside.
3. Cut toasted waffles into cubes.

4. Layer bacon and waffle cubes with cheese and green onions in a 3½-quart slow cooker.
5. Drain skillet, discarding bacon fat; do not wipe out.
6. Put the milk plus cream cheese in skillet; cook over low heat, stirring frequently.
7. Remove, then beat in eggs, one at a time, until smooth.
8. Stir in dry mustard, then pour into a slow cooker.
9. Cover and cook on low within 4–5 hours, until eggs are set.
10. Serve with warmed maple syrup, if desired.

Nutrition:

- Calories: 382
- Carbs: 25 g
- Fat: 22 g
- Protein: 21 g

Honey Apple Bread Pudding

Preparation time:

15 minutes

Cooking time:

4 hours & 35 minutes

Servings:

4 people

Ingredients:

- 2 apples, chopped
- ¼ cup apple juice
- cup brown sugar
- ¼ cup honey
- 2 tablespoons butter, melted
- 4 eggs, beaten
- cup whole milk
- 1 teaspoon vanilla
- ½ teaspoon cinnamon
- 8 slices raisin swirl bread
- ½ cup raisins

Directions:

1. In a medium saucepan, combine apples with apple juice.

2. Bring to a simmer; simmer for 5 minutes, stirring frequently.
3. Remove, then set aside within 10 minutes. Drain apples, reserving juice.
4. Mix brown sugar, honey, and butter in a small bowl; set aside.
5. In a large bowl, combine reserved apple juice, eggs, milk, vanilla, and cinnamon; beat well and set aside.
6. Cut bread slices into cubes. In the slow cooker, layer the bread cubes, raisins, apples, and the brown sugar mixture.
7. Repeat layers. Pour egg mixture overall.
8. Cover and cook on high within 3 to 4 hours and 30 minutes, until pudding is set.
9. Let cool within 30 minutes, then serve.

Nutrition:

- Calories: 312
- Carbs: 41 g
- Fat: 15 g
- Protein: 7 g

Sausage Rolls

Preparation time:

15 minutes

Cooking time:

9 hours & 6 minutes

Servings:

4 people

Ingredients:

- ¾ cup soft bread crumbs
- 1 egg, beaten
- ¼ cup brown sugar
- ¼ cup applesauce
- ½ teaspoon salt
- 1 teaspoon pepper
- ½ teaspoon dried marjoram leaves
- 1½-pounds mild bulk pork sausage
- 2 tablespoons butter
- ¼ cup honey
- ¼ cup chicken broth

Directions:

1. In a large bowl, combine crumbs, egg, brown sugar, applesauce, salt, pepper, and marjoram.

2. Mix well. Stir in sausage.
3. Shape into rolls 3" × 1". Dissolve the butter over medium heat in a large skillet.
4. Add sausage rolls, about 8 at a time, and cook until browned on all sides, about 5–6 minutes.
5. As rolls cook, drain on paper towels, then place into the 3-quart slow cooker.
6. In a small bowl, combine honey and chicken broth and mix well.
7. Pour over sausage rolls in a slow cooker.
8. Cook on low within 8–9 hours or until sausage rolls are thoroughly cooked, to 165°F on a meat thermometer.
9. Remove from slow cooker with a slotted spoon to serve.

Nutrition:

- Calories: 102
- Carbs: 7 g
- Fat: 0 g
- Protein: 7 g

Breakfast Pitas

Preparation time:

15 minutes

Cooking time:

7-8 hours & 5 minutes

Servings:

4 people

Ingredients:

- 2 tablespoons butter
- 1 onion, chopped
- 2 cloves garlic, chopped
- 8 eggs, beaten
- ½ teaspoon salt
- 1 teaspoon pepper
- ½ cup of salsa
- 1 cup shredded pepper jack cheese
- 4 pita bread
- 2 tablespoons chopped parsley

Directions:

1. Oiled 2-quart slow cooker with nonstick cooking spray.

2. In a small skillet, melt butter over medium heat.
3. Put the onion plus garlic; cook and stir until tender, about 5 minutes.
4. Remove from heat.
5. Mix eggs, salt, and pepper and beat well in a large bowl.
6. Stir in onion mixture, salsa, and cheese. Pour into the slow cooker.
7. Cover and cook on low within 7–8 hours.
8. In the morning, stir the mixture in a slow cooker.
9. Split pita bread and fill with egg mixture; top with parsley and serve immediately.

Nutrition:

- Calories: 200
- Carbs: 14g
- Fat: 1g
- Protein: 6g

Oregano Salsa

Preparation time:

10 minutes

Cooking time:

7 hours

Servings:

4 people

Ingredients:

- 3 cups eggplant, cubed
- 4 garlic cloves, minced
- 6 oz. green olives, pitted and sliced
- 1 and ½ cups tomatoes, chopped
- 2 teaspoons balsamic vinegar
- 1 tablespoon oregano, chopped
- Black pepper to the taste

Directions:

1. In your slow cooker, mix tomatoes with eggplant, green olives, garlic, vinegar, oregano, and pepper, toss, cover, cook on low for 7 hours, divide into small bowls and serve as an appetizer.

Nutrition:

- Calories: 78
- Fat: 3.6 g
- Carbs: 11.2 g
- Protein: 2 g

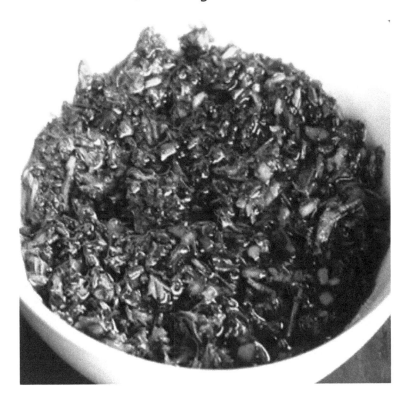

Smoked Paprika Cauliflower Spread

Preparation time:

10 minutes

Cooking time:

7 hours

Servings:

4 people

Ingredients:

- 2 cups cauliflower florets
- 1 cup of coconut milk
- 1/3 cup cashews, chopped
- 2 and ½ cups of water
- 1 cup turnips, chopped
- 1 teaspoon garlic powder
- ¼ teaspoon smoked paprika
- ¼ teaspoon mustard powder

Directions:

1. In your slow cooker, mix cauliflower with cashews, turnips, and water, stir, cover, cook on low for 7 hours, drain, transfer to a blender, add milk, garlic powder, paprika, and mustard powder, blend well, and serve.

Nutrition:

- Calories: 228
- Fat: 19.7 g
- Carbs: 12.4 g
- Protein: 4.6 g

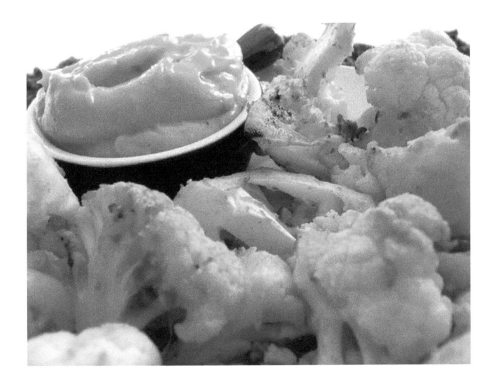

French Style Salad

Preparation time:

10 minutes

Cooking time:

9 hours

Servings:

4 people

Ingredients:

- 6 oz. canned tomato paste, no-salt-added
- 2 tomatoes, cut into medium wedges
- 2 yellow onions, chopped
- 1 eggplant, sliced
- 4 zucchinis, sliced
- 2 green bell peppers, cut into medium strips
- 2 garlic cloves, minced
- 2 tablespoons parsley, chopped
- 3 tablespoons olive oil
- 1 teaspoon oregano, dried
- 1 tablespoon basil, chopped
- A pinch of black pepper

Directions:

1. In your slow cooker, mix oil with onions, eggplant, zucchinis, garlic, bell peppers, tomato paste, tomatoes, basil, oregano, and pepper, cover, and cook on low for 9 hours.
2. Add parsley, toss, divide into small bowls and serve warm as an appetizer.

Nutrition:

- Calories: 161
- Fat: 7.8g
- Carbs: 22.8g
- Protein: 4.9g

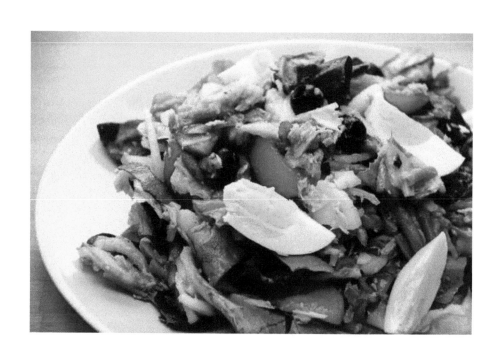

Stevia and Bulgur Salad

Preparation time:

10 minutes

Cooking time:

12 hours

Servings:

4 people

Ingredients:

- 2 cups white mushrooms, sliced
- 14 oz. canned kidney beans, no-salt-added, drained
- 14 oz. canned pinto beans, no-salt-added, drained
- 2 cups yellow onion, chopped
- 1 cup low sodium veggie stock
- 1 cup strong coffee
- ¾ cup bulgur, soaked and drained
- ½ cup red bell pepper, chopped
- 2 garlic cloves, minced
- 2 tablespoons stevia
- 2 tablespoons chili powder
- 1 tablespoon cocoa powder
- 1 teaspoon oregano, dried

- 2 teaspoons cumin, ground
- Black pepper to the taste

Directions:

1. In your slow cooker, mix mushrooms with bulgur, onion, bell pepper, stock, garlic, coffee, kidney and pinto beans, stevia, chili powder, cocoa, oregano, cumin, and pepper, stir gently, cover, and cook on low for 12 hours.
2. Divide the mix into small bowls and serve cold as an appetizer.

Nutrition:

- Calories: 837
- Fat: 4.2 g
- Carbs: 162 g
- Protein: 49.9 g

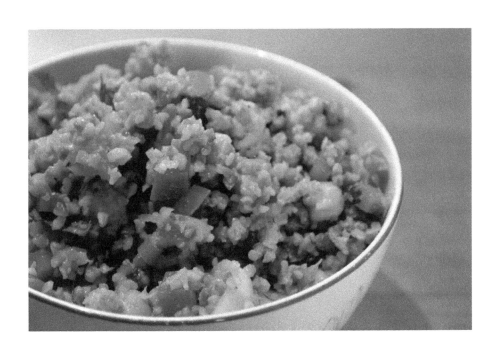

Parmesan Stuffed Mushrooms

Preparation time:

10 minutes

Cooking time:

5 hours

Servings:

4 people

Ingredients:

- 20 mushrooms, stems removed
- 2 cups basil, chopped
- 1 cup tomato sauce, no-salt-added
- 2 tablespoons parsley, chopped
- ¼ cup low-fat parmesan, grated
- 1 and ½ cups whole wheat breadcrumbs
- 1 tablespoon garlic, minced
- ¼ cup low-fat butter, melted
- 2 teaspoons lemon juice
- 1 tablespoon olive oil

Directions:

1. In a bowl, mix butter with breadcrumbs and parsley, stir well, and leave aside.

2. In your blender, mix basil with oil, parmesan, garlic, and lemon juice and pulse well.
3. Stuff mushrooms with this mix, pour the tomato sauce on top, sprinkle breadcrumbs mix at the end, and cook in the slow cooker on low for 5 hours.
4. Arrange mushrooms on a platter and serve.

Nutrition:

- Calories: 51
- Fat: 1.1 g
- Carbs: 9 g
- Protein: 2.2 g

Garlic and Tomato Appetizer

Preparation time:

10 minutes

Cooking time:

2 hours

Servings:

4 people

Ingredients:

- 2 teaspoons olive oil
- 8 tomatoes, chopped
- 1 garlic clove, minced
- ¼ cup basil, chopped
- 4 Italian whole wheat bread slices, toasted
- 3 tablespoons low-sodium veggie stock
- Black pepper to the taste

Directions:

1. In your slow cooker, mix tomatoes with basil, garlic, oil, veggie stock, and black pepper, stir, cover, cook on high within 2 hours and then leave aside to cool down.
2. Divide this mix on the toasted bread and serve as an appetizer.

Nutrition:

- Calories: 158
- Fat: 4.1 g
- Carbs: 26.3 g
- Protein: 5.9 g

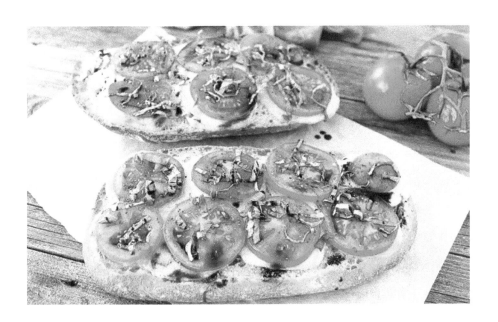

Tahini Dip

Preparation time:

10 minutes

Cooking time:

3 hours

Servings:

4 people

Ingredients:

- ½ pound cauliflower florets
- 1 teaspoon avocado oil
- 1 tablespoon ginger, grated
- 1 cup coconut cream
- 3 garlic cloves, minced
- Black pepper to the taste
- 1 tablespoon basil, chopped
- 1 tablespoon tahini paste
- 1 tablespoon lime juice

Directions:

1. In your slow cooker, combine the cauliflower with the oil, ginger, and the other ingredients, cook on low within 3 hours.

2. Transfer to your blender, pulse well, divide into bowls and serve.

Nutrition:

- Calories: 217
- Fat: 18.1 g
- Carbs: 13.3 g
- Protein: 3.7 g

Lime Juice Snack

Preparation time:

10 minutes

Cooking time:

2 hours

Servings:

4 people

Ingredients:

- 1 pineapple, peeled and cut into medium sticks
- 2 tablespoons stevia
- 1 tablespoon olive oil
- 1 tablespoon lime juice
- 1 tablespoon lime zest, grated
- 1 teaspoon cinnamon powder
- ¼ teaspoon cloves, ground

Directions:

1. In a bowl, mix lime juice with stevia, oil, cinnamon, and cloves and whisk well.
2. Add the pineapple sticks to your slow cooker, add lime mix, toss, cover, and cook on high for 2 hours.

3. Serve the pineapple sticks as a snack with lime zest sprinkled on top.

Nutrition:

- Calories: 26
- Fat: 1.8 g
- Carbs: 6.1 g
- Protein: 0.1 g

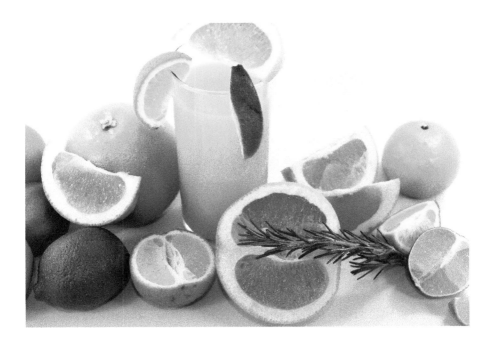

Cumin Hummus

Preparation time:

10 minutes

Cooking time:

5 hours

Servings:

4 people

Ingredients:

- 1 cup chickpeas, soaked overnight and drained
- 2 garlic cloves
- ¾ cup green onions, chopped
- 1 tablespoon olive oil
- 2 tablespoons sherry vinegar
- 3 cups of water
- 1 teaspoon cumin, ground

Directions:

1. Put the water in your slow cooker, add chickpeas and garlic, cover, and cook on low for 5 hours.
2. Drain chickpeas, transfer them to your blender, add ½ cup of the cooking liquid,

green onions, vinegar, oil, cilantro, and cumin, blend well, divide into bowls and serve.

Nutrition:

- Calories: 150
- Fat: 4.5 g
- Carbs: 22.3 g
- Protein: 6.8 g

Peppercorns Asparagus

Preparation time:

10 minutes

Cooking time:

2 hours

Servings:

4 people

Ingredients:

- 3 cups asparagus spears, halved
- 3 garlic cloves, sliced
- 1 tablespoon dill
- ¼ cup white wine vinegar
- ¼ cup apple cider vinegar
- 2 cloves
- 1 cup of water
- ¼ teaspoon red pepper flakes
- 8 black peppercorns
- 1 teaspoon coriander seeds

Directions:

1. In your slow cooker, mix the asparagus with the cider vinegar, white vinegar, dill, cloves, water, garlic, pepper flakes, peppercorns, and

coriander, cover, and cook on high for 2
hours.

2. Drain asparagus, transfer it to bowls, and
   serve as a snack.

Nutrition:

- Calories: 20
- Fat: 0.1 g
- Carbs: 3.6 g
- Protein: 1.7 g

Light Shrimp Salad

Preparation time:

10 minutes

Cooking time:

5 hours and 30 minutes

Servings:

4 people

Ingredients:

- 1 cup tomato, chopped
- ¼ pound shrimp, peeled, deveined, and chopped
- 1 cup canned black beans, no-salt-added, drained and rinsed
- 1 cup cucumber, chopped
- 2 teaspoons cumin, ground
- 2 tablespoons olive oil
- ½ cup red onion, chopped
- Zest and juice of 2 limes
- Zest and juice of 2 lemons
- 2 tablespoons garlic, minced
- ¼ cup cilantro, chopped

Directions:

1. In a bowl, mix lime juice and lemon juice with shrimp and toss.
2. Grease the slow cooker with the oil, add black beans, tomato, onion, garlic, and cumin, cover, and cook on low within 5 hours.
3. Add shrimp, cover, cook on low for 30 minutes, more, transfer everything to a bowl, add cucumber and cilantro, toss, leave aside to cool down, divide between small bowls and serve as an appetizer.

Nutrition:

- Calories: 153
- Fat: 4.4 g
- Carbs: 21.4 g
- Protein: 9.3 g

Mushroom Salsa with Pumpkin Seeds

Preparation time:

10 minutes

Cooking time:

3 hours

Servings:

4 people

Ingredients:

- 1-pound white mushrooms, sliced
- 1 cup cherry tomatoes, halved
- 1 cup black olives, pitted and sliced
- 1 tablespoon olive oil
- Juice of 1 lime
- 2 tablespoons parsley, chopped
- 2 tablespoons pumpkin seeds
- 1 tablespoon basil, chopped
- 1 tablespoon balsamic vinegar

Directions:

1. In a slow cooker, combine the mushrooms with the tomatoes, olives, and the other ingredients, cook on low within 3 hours.

2. Divide the salsa into bowls and serve as an appetizer.

Nutrition:

- Calories: 129
- Fat: 9.5 g
- Carbs: 9.4 g
- Protein: 5.4 g

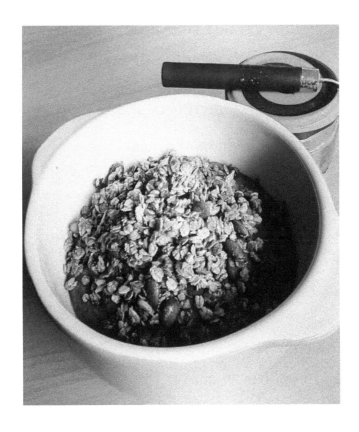

Onion Chickpeas Dip

Preparation time:

10 minutes

Cooking time:

2 hours

Servings:

4 people

Ingredients:

- 2 cups canned chickpeas, no-salt-added, drained and rinsed
- 1 cup red bell pepper, sliced
- 1 teaspoon onion powder
- 1 tablespoon lemon juice
- 1 teaspoon garlic powder
- 1 tablespoon olive oil
- 2 tablespoons white sesame seeds
- A pinch of cayenne pepper
- 1 and ¼ teaspoons cumin, ground

Directions:

1. In your slow cooker, mix red bell pepper with oil, sesame seeds, chickpeas, lemon juice,

garlic and onion powder, cayenne pepper, cumin, cover, and cook on high for 2 hours.

2. Transfer this mix to your blender, pulse well, divide into serving bowls and serve cold.

Nutrition:

- Calories: 143
- Fat: 3.8 g
- Carbs: 21.6 g
- Protein: 6.8 g

Garlic and Beans Spread

Preparation time:

10 minutes

Cooking time:

6 hours

Servings:

4 people

Ingredients:

- 15 oz. canned white beans, no-salt-added, drained and rinsed
- 8 garlic cloves, roasted
- 1 cup low-sodium veggie stock
- 2 tablespoons lemon juice
- 2 tablespoons olive oil

Directions:

1. In your blender, mix beans with oil, stock, garlic, and lemon juice, cover the slow cooker, cook on low for 6 hours, transfer to your blender, pulse well, divide into bowls and serve as a snack.

Nutrition:

- Calories: 214
- Fat: 4 g
- Carbs: 33.2 g
- Protein: 12.9 g

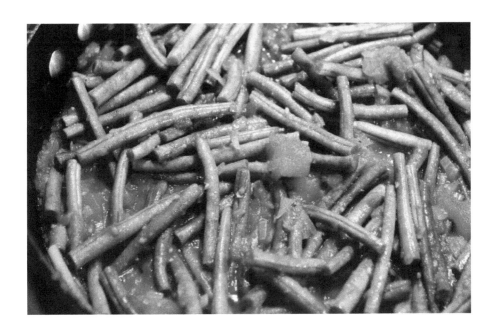

Sour Cream Dip

Preparation time:

20 minutes

Cooking time:

2 hours

Servings:

4 people

Ingredients:

- 1 bunch spinach leaves, roughly chopped
- ¾ cup low-fat sour cream
- 1 scallion, sliced
- 2 tablespoons mint leaves, chopped
- Black pepper to the taste

Directions:

1. In your slow cooker, mix the spinach with the scallion, mint, cream, and black pepper, cover, cook on high within 2 hours, stir well, divide into bowls and serve.

Nutrition:

- Calories: 121

- Fat: 9.7 g
- Carbs: 6.3 g
- Protein: 4 g

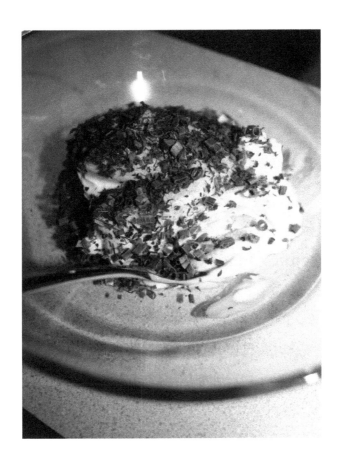

Simple Meatballs

Preparation time:

10 minutes

Cooking time:

8 hours

Servings:

16 meatballs

Ingredients:

- 1 and ½ pounds beef, ground
- 1 egg, whisked
- 16 oz. canned tomatoes, crushed
- 14 oz. canned tomato puree
- ¼ cup parsley, chopped
- 2 garlic cloves, minced
- 1 yellow onion, chopped
- Black pepper to the taste

Directions:

1. In a bowl, mix beef with egg, parsley, garlic, black pepper, and onion and stir well.
2. Shape 16 meatballs, place them in your slow cooker, add tomato puree and crushed

tomatoes on top, cover, and cook on low
within 8 hours.

3. Arrange them on a platter and serve.
4. Enjoy!

Nutrition:

- Calories: 160
- Fat: 5 g
- Carbs: 10 g
- Protein: 7 g

Tasty Chicken Wings

Preparation time:

10 minutes

Cooking time:

3 hours

Servings:

6

Ingredients:

- 2 tablespoons garlic, minced
- 2 and ¼ cups pineapple juice
- 3 tablespoons coconut aminos
- 2 tablespoons tapioca flour
- 1 tablespoon ginger, minced
- 1 teaspoon sesame oil
- A pinch of sea salt
- 3 pounds of chicken wings
- A few red pepper flakes, crushed
- 2 tablespoons 5 spice powder
- Sesame seeds, toasted for serving
- Chopped cilantro, for serving

Directions:

1. Put 2 cups pineapple juice in your slow cooker, add sesame oil, a pinch of salt, coconut aminos, ginger, and garlic, and whisk well.
2. In a bowl, mix tapioca flour with the rest of the pineapple juice, whisk, and add to your slow cooker.
3. Whisk everything and then add chicken wings.
4. Season them with pepper flakes and 5 spice, toss everything, cover and cook on high for 3 hours.
5. Transfer chicken wings to a platter and sprinkle cilantro and sesame seeds on top.
6. Transfer sauce from the slow cooker to a pot and heat it for 2 minutes over medium-high heat.
7. Whisk well, pour into small bowls, and serve your wings with it.
8. Enjoy!

Nutrition:

- Calories: 200
- Fat: 4 g
- Carbs: 9 g
- Protein: 20 g

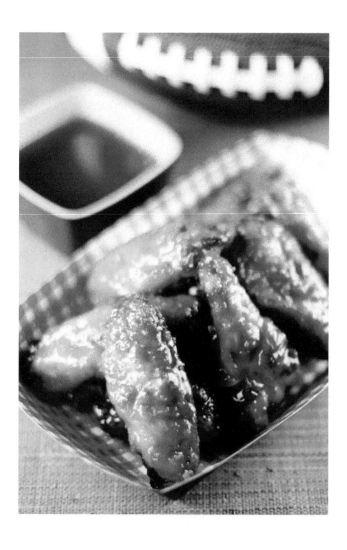

Chicken Spread

Preparation time:

10 minutes

Cooking time:

2 hours

Servings:

4 people

Ingredients:

- 12 oz. chicken breasts, skinless, boneless, cooked and shredded
- 10 oz. coconut cream
- 1 cup of coconut milk
- 1 cup hot sauce
- A pinch of salt and black pepper
- ½ teaspoon garlic powder
- ¼ cup scallions, chopped
- ½ teaspoon onion powder

Directions:

1. Mix the chicken with the cream, coconut milk, hot sauce, salt, pepper, garlic powder, scallions, and onion powder in your slow cooker, toss, cover, cook on low for 2 hours,

stir again, divide into bowls and serve as a spread.

2. Enjoy!

Nutrition:

- Calories: 214
- Fat: 4 g
- Carbs: 16 g
- Protein: 17 g

Different Chicken Dip

Preparation time:

10 minutes

Cooking time:

3 hours and 30 minutes

Servings:

4 people

Ingredients:

- 1 yellow onion, chopped
- 2 teaspoons olive oil
- 1 red bell pepper, chopped
- 3 cups rotisserie chicken, cooked and shredded
- 12 oz. coconut cream
- ½ cup chili sauce
- 2 tablespoons chives, chopped

Directions:

1. Heat-up a pan with the oil over medium-high heat, add the onion, stir, cook for 5 minutes and transfer to your slow cooker.
2. Add bell pepper, cream, chicken, chili sauce, chives, toss, cover, cook on low for 3 hours

and 30 minutes, divide into bowls and serve
as a party dip.

3. Enjoy!

Nutrition:

- Calories: 251
- Fat: 5 g
- Carbs: 17 g
- Protein: 18 g

Carrot Dip

Preparation time:

10 minutes

Cooking time:

5 hours

Servings:

4

Ingredients:

- 2-pound carrots, peeled and chopped
- ¼ cup olive oil
- 2 teaspoons cumin, ground
- A pinch of salt and black pepper
- 4 garlic cloves, minced
- ½ cup veggie stock

Directions:

1. Grease your slow cooker with half of the oil, add carrots, cumin, salt, pepper, garlic, and stock, toss, cover, cook on low for 5 hours, transfer to your blender, add the rest of the oil, pulse well, divide into bowls and serve.
2. Enjoy!

Nutrition:

- Calories: 211
- Fat: 6 g
- Carbs: 13 g
- Protein: 7 g

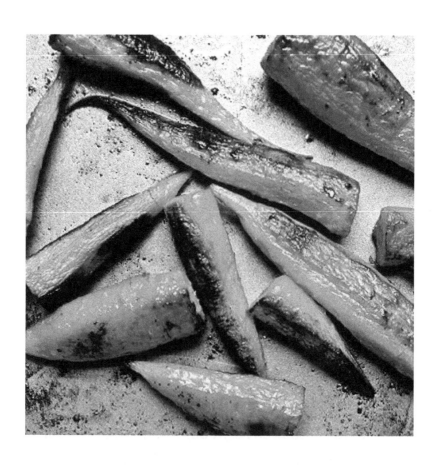

Pepperoni Dip

Preparation time:

10 minutes

Cooking time:

1 hour

Servings:

4 people

Ingredients:

- 13 oz. coconut cream
- 8 oz. pepperoni, sliced
- A pinch of black pepper

Directions:

1. In your slow cooker, combine the cream with the pepperoni and black pepper, cover, cook on low for 1 hour, stir, divide into bowls and serve.
2. Enjoy!

Nutrition:

- Calories: 231
- Fat: 4 g

- Carbs: 16 g
- Protein: 11 g

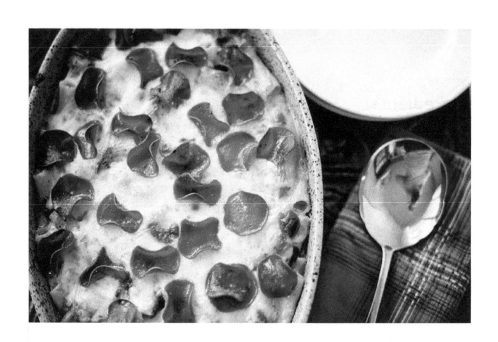

Eggplant Spread

Preparation time:

10 minutes

Cooking time:

1 hour and 30 minutes

Servings:

4 people

Ingredients:

- 2 pounds eggplants, peeled and cubed
- 1 tablespoon sesame paste
- 3 tablespoons lemon juice
- 1 garlic clove, minced
- ¼ teaspoon liquid smoke
- ½ teaspoon olive oil
- Handful parsley, chopped

Directions:

1. In your slow cooker, combine the eggplants with the sesame paste, lemon juice, garlic, liquid smoke, oil, parsley, toss, cover, cook on high for 1 hour and 30 minutes, pulse using an immersion blender, and serve.
2. Enjoy!

Nutrition:

- Calories: 211
- Fat: 4 g
- Carbs: 15 g
- Protein: 7 g

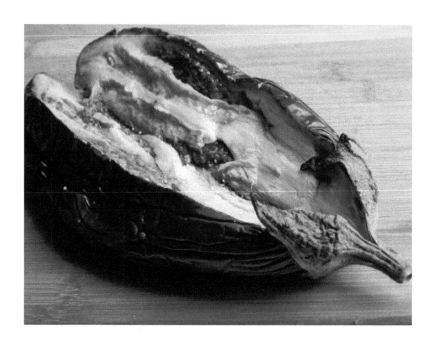

Jalapeno Poppers

Preparation time:

10 minutes

Cooking time:

3 hours

Servings:

4 people

Ingredients:

- ½ pound chorizo, chopped
- 10 jalapenos, tops cut off and deseeded
- 1 small white onion, chopped
- ½ pound beef, ground
- ¼ teaspoon garlic powder
- 1 tablespoon maple syrup
- 1 tablespoon mustard
- 1/3 cup water

Directions:

1. Mix the beef with chorizo, garlic powder, and onion in a bowl.
2. Stuff your jalapenos with the mix and put them in your slow cooker.

3. Put the water, cover, and cook on high within 3 hours.

4. Move the jalapeno poppers to a lined baking sheet. In a bowl, mix maple syrup with mustard and whisk well.

5. Brush poppers with this mix, introduce in the preheated broiler and cook for 10 minutes.

6. Arrange on a platter and serve.

7. Enjoy!

Nutrition:

- Calories: 200
- Fat: 2 g
- Carbs: 8 g
- Protein: 3 g

Fish Sticks

Preparation time:

10 minutes

Cooking time:

2 hours

Servings:

4 people

Ingredients:

- 2 eggs, whisked
- 1-pound cod fillets, cut into medium strips
- 1 and ½ cups almond flour
- A pinch of sea salt
- Black pepper to the taste
- ½ cup tapioca flour
- ¼ teaspoon paprika
- Cooking spray

Directions:

1. In a bowl, mix almond flour, salt, pepper, tapioca, and paprika and stir.
2. Put the eggs in another bowl.
3. Dip fish sticks in the eggs and then dredge in the flour mix.

4. Spray your slow cooker with cooking spray and arrange fish sticks in it—cover and cook on high within 2 hours.
5. Arrange on a platter and serve.
6. Enjoy!

Nutrition:

- Calories: 200
- Fat: 2g
- Carbs: 7 g
- Protein: 12 g

Spicy Pecans

Preparation time:

10 minutes

Cooking time:

2 hours and 15 minutes

Servings:

4 people

Ingredients:

- 1-pound pecans halved
- 2 tablespoons olive oil
- 1 teaspoon basil, dried
- 1 tablespoon chili powder
- 1 teaspoon oregano, dried
- ¼ teaspoon garlic powder
- 1 teaspoon thyme, dried
- ½ teaspoon onion powder
- A pinch of cayenne pepper

Directions:

1. In your slow cooker, mix pecans with oil, basil, chili powder, oregano, garlic powder, onion powder, thyme, and cayenne and toss to coat.
2. Cover and cook on high within 15 minutes.

3. Switch slow cooker to low and cook for 2 hours.
4. Serve as a snack.
5. Enjoy!

Nutrition:

- Calories: 78
- Fat: 3 g
- Carbs: 9 g
- Protein: 2 g

Sausage Appetizer

Preparation time:

10 minutes

Cooking time:

2 hours

Servings:

15 sausages

Ingredients:

- 2 pounds sausages, sliced
- 18 oz. unsweetened apple jelly
- 9 oz. Dijon mustard

Directions:

1. Place sausage slices in your slow cooker, add apple jelly and mustard and toss to coat well.
2. Cover and cook on low within 2 hours, stirring every 20 minutes.
3. Arrange sausage slices on a platter and serve as an appetizer.
4. Enjoy!

Nutrition:

- Calories: 140
- Fat: 3 g
- Carbs: 9 g
- Protein: 10 g

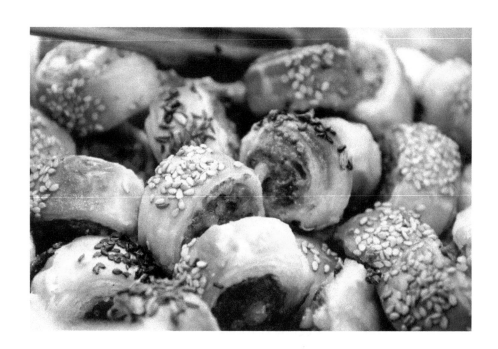

Asparagus Spread

Preparation time:

10 minutes

Cooking time:

2 hours and 30 minutes

Servings:

4 people

Ingredients:

- 1 bunch asparagus, roughly chopped
- 4 garlic cloves, minced
- 5 oz. coconut cream
- ½ teaspoon garlic powder
- ½ teaspoon red pepper flakes
- ¼ teaspoon onion powder
- ¼ teaspoon paprika
- 6 oz. baby spinach
- 2 teaspoons olive oil
- ½ cup veggie stock

Directions:

1. In your slow cooker, combine the asparagus with the garlic, cream, garlic powder, pepper flakes, onion powder, paprika, spinach, stock,

and oil, toss, cover, cook on low for 2 hours and 30 minutes, pulse using an immersion blender and serve.

2. Enjoy!

Nutrition:

- Calories: 221
- Fat: 4 g
- Carbs: 16 g
- Protein: 8 g

Broccoli Dip

Preparation time:

10 minutes

Cooking time:

2 hours

Servings:

4 people

Ingredients:

- 1 yellow onion, chopped
- 6 bacon slices, cooked and chopped
- 2 garlic cloves, minced
- ¼ teaspoon red pepper flakes, crushed
- 4 cups broccoli florets, chopped
- 8 oz. coconut cream
- 1 tablespoon scallions, chopped
- ½ cup avocado mayonnaise
- ½ cup of coconut milk
- A pinch of salt and black pepper

Directions:

1. In your slow cooker, combine the onion with the bacon, garlic, pepper flakes, broccoli, cream, scallions, mayo, milk, salt and pepper,

stir, cover, cook on low for 2 hours, stir again really well, divide into bowls and serve.

2. Enjoy!

Nutrition:

- Calories: 261
- Fat: 11 g
- Carbs: 8 g
- Protein: 12 g

Crab and Onion Dip

Preparation time:

10 minutes

Cooking time:

4 hours

Servings:

4 people

Ingredients:

- 24 oz. coconut cream
- 12 oz. canned crabmeat, drained
- ¼ cup of coconut milk
- 4 green onions, chopped
- 2 teaspoons horseradish, prepared
- A pinch of salt and black pepper

Directions:

1. In your slow cooker, combine the cream with the crabmeat, milk, onions, salt, pepper, and horseradish, stir, cover, cook on low for 4 hours, divide into bowls and serve.
2. Enjoy!

Nutrition:

- Calories: 167
- Fat: 8 g
- Carbs: 2 g
- Protein: 7 g

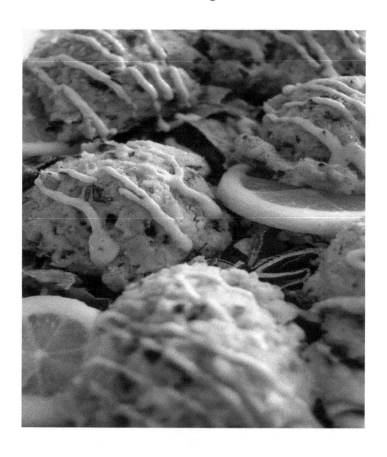

Spinach and Bacon Dip

Preparation time:

10 minutes

Cooking time:

2 hours

Servings:

4 people

Ingredients:

- 16 oz. coconut cream
- 1 cup of coconut milk
- 15 oz. canned artichokes, drained and chopped
- 10 oz. spinach, chopped
- 2 tomatoes, chopped
- ½ cup bacon, cooked and crumbled
- 4 green onions, chopped

Directions:

1. In your slow cooker, combine the cream with coconut milk, spinach, artichokes, tomatoes, and green onions, stir, cover, cook on low for 2 hours, divide into bowls, sprinkle bacon on top, and serve.

2. Enjoy!

Nutrition:

- Calories: 200
- Fat: 6 g
- Carbs: 9 g
- Protein: 6 g

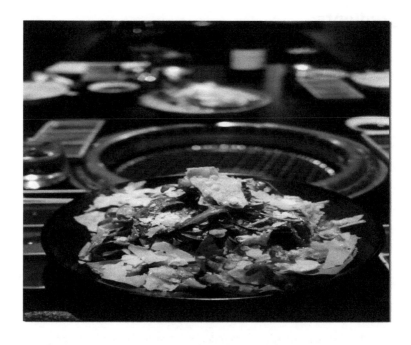

Bean Pesto Dip

Preparation time:

15 minutes

Cooking time:

6 hours

Servings:

4 people

Ingredients:

- 10 oz. refried beans
- 1 tbsp pesto sauce
- 1 tsp salt
- 7 oz. Cheddar cheese, shredded
- 1 tsp paprika
- 1 cup of salsa
- 4 tbsp sour cream
- 2-oz. cream cheese
- 1 tsp dried dill

Directions:

1. Mix pesto with salt, salsa, sour cream, dill, beans, cheese, paprika, and cream cheese in the slow cooker.

2. Put the cooker's lid on and set the cooking time to 6 hours on low.
3. Blend the mixture using a hand blender.
4. Serve fresh.

Nutrition:

- Calories: 102
- Fat: 6.3 g
- Carbs: 7.43 g
- Protein: 5 g

Cheesy Chili Pepper Dip

Preparation time:

15 minutes

Cooking time:

9 hours

Servings:

4 people

Ingredients:

- 4 chili pepper, sliced and deseeded
- 7 oz. Monterey cheese
- 3 tbsp cream cheese
- 1 tbsp onion powder
- 3 tbsp dried dill
- 3 oz. butter
- 1 tbsp cornstarch
- 1 tbsp flour
- ¼ tsp salt

Directions:

1. Add chili peppers to a blender and add salt, butter, onion powder, and dill.
2. Blend the chili peppers well, then transfer to the slow cooker.

3. Stir in flour, cornstarch, cream cheese, and
4. Monterey cheese.
5. Put the cooker's lid on and set the cooking time to 6 hours on low.
6. Serve.

Nutrition:

- Calories: 212
- Fat: 18.2 g
- Carbs: 6.06 g
- Protein: 8 g

Creamy Mushroom Spread

Preparation time:

15 minutes

Cooking time:

4 hours

Servings:

2 people

Ingredients:

- 1-pound mushrooms, sliced
- 3 garlic cloves, minced
- 1 cup heavy cream
- 2 teaspoons smoked paprika
- Salt and black pepper to the taste
- 2 tablespoons parsley, chopped

Directions:

1. In your slow cooker, mix the mushrooms with the garlic and the other ingredients, whisk, cook on low within 4 hours.
2. Whisk, divide into bowls, and serve as a party spread.

Nutrition:

- Calories: 300
- Fat: 6 g
- Carbs: 16 g
- Protein: 6 g

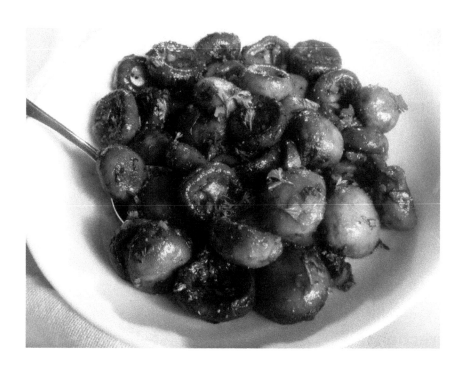

Pork Tostadas

Preparation time:

15 minutes

Cooking time:

4 hours

Servings:

4 people

Ingredients:

- 4 lbs. pork shoulder, boneless and cubed
- Salt and black pepper to the taste
- 2 cups coca cola
- 1/3 cup brown sugar
- ½ cup hot sauce
- 2 tsp chili powder
- 2 tbsp tomato paste
- ¼ tsp cumin, ground
- 1 cup enchilada sauce
- Corn tortillas, toasted for a few minutes in the oven
- Mexican cheese, shredded for serving
- 4 shredded lettuce leaves, for serving
- Salsa
- Guacamole for serving

Directions:

1. Add cup coke, salsa, sugar, chili powder, cumin, pork, hot sauce, and tomato paste to the slow cooker.
2. Put the cooker's lid on and set the cooking time to 4 hours on low.
3. Drain the cooked pork and shred it finely.
4. Mix well the shredded pork with enchilada sauce and remaining coke.
5. Divide the pork into the tortillas and top it with lettuce leaves, guacamole, and Mexican cheese.
6. Serve.

Nutrition:

- Calories: 162
- Fat: 3g
- Carbs: 12 g
- Protein: 5 g

BBQ Chicken Dip

Preparation time:

15 minutes

Cooking time:

1 hour and 30 minutes

Servings:

4 people

Ingredients:

- 1 and ½ cups BBQ sauce
- 1 small red onion, chopped
- 24 oz. cream cheese, cubed
- 2 cups rotisserie chicken, shredded
- 3 bacon slices, cooked and crumbled
- 1 plum tomato, chopped
- ½ cup cheddar cheese, shredded
- 1 tablespoon green onions, chopped

Directions:

1. In your slow cooker, mix BBQ sauce with onion, cream cheese, rotisserie chicken, bacon, tomato, cheddar, and green onions, stir, cover, and cook on low for 1 hour and 30 minutes.

2. Divide into bowls and serve.

Nutrition:

- Calories: 251
- Fat: 4 g
- Carbs: 10 g
- Protein: 4 g

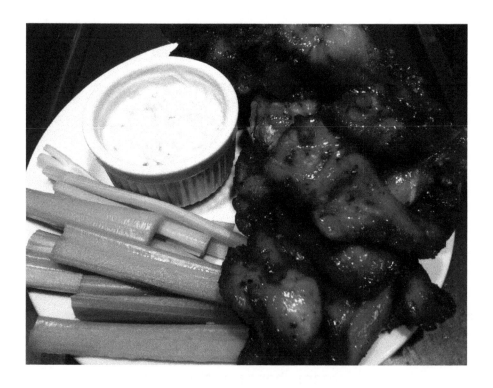

Lemon Shrimp Dip

Preparation time:

15 minutes

Cooking time:

2 hours

Servings:

2 people

Ingredients:

- 3 oz. cream cheese, soft
- ½ cup heavy cream
- 1-pound shrimp, peeled, deveined, and chopped
- ½ tablespoon balsamic vinegar
- 2 tablespoons mayonnaise
- ½ tablespoon lemon juice
- A pinch of salt and black pepper
- 2 oz. mozzarella, shredded
- 1 tablespoon parsley, chopped

Directions:

1. In your slow cooker, mix the cream cheese with the shrimp, heavy cream, and the other

ingredients, whisk, put the lid on and cook on low for 2 hours.

2. Divide into bowls and serve.

Nutrition:

- Calories: 342
- Fat: 4 g
- Carbs: 7 g
- Protein: 10 g

Zucchini Sticks

Preparation time:

15 minutes

Cooking time:

2 hours

Servings:

13 sticks

Ingredients:

- 9 oz. green zucchini, cut into thick sticks
- 4 oz. Parmesan, grated
- 1 egg
- 1 tsp salt
- 1 tsp ground white pepper
- 1 tsp olive oil
- 2 tbsp milk

Directions:

1. Grease the base of your slow cooker with olive oil. Whisk egg with milk, white pepper, and salt in a bowl.
2. Dip the prepared zucchini sticks in the egg mixture, then place them in the slow cooker.

3. Put the cooker's lid on and set the cooking time to 2 hours on high.
4. Spread the cheese over the zucchini sticks evenly.
5. Put the cooker's lid on and set the cooking time to 2 hours on high.
6. Serve.

Nutrition:

- Calories: 51
- Fat: 1.7 g
- Carbs: 4.62 g
- Protein: 5 g

Chicken Cordon Bleu Dip

Preparation time:

15 minutes

Cooking time:

1 hour & 30 minutes

Servings:

4 people

Ingredients:

- 16 oz. cream cheese
- 2 chicken breasts, baked and shredded
- 1 cup cheddar cheese, shredded
- 1 cup Swiss cheese, shredded
- 3 garlic cloves, minced
- 6 oz. ham, chopped
- 2 tablespoons green onions
- Salt and black pepper to the taste

Directions:

1. In your slow cooker, mix cream cheese with chicken, cheddar cheese, Swiss cheese, garlic, ham, green onions, salt, and pepper, stir, cover, and cook on low for 1 hour and 30 minutes.

2. Serve.

Nutrition:

- Calories: 243
- Fat: 5 g
- Carbs: 15 g
- Protein: 3 g

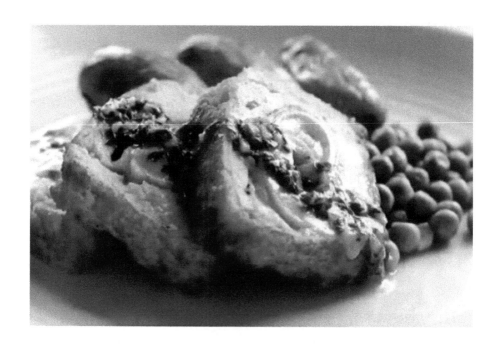

Eggplant Zucchini Dip

Preparation time:

15 minutes

Cooking time:

4 hours & 5 minutes

Servings:

4 people

Ingredients:

- 1 eggplant
- 1 zucchini, chopped
- 2 tbsp olive oil
- 2 tbsp balsamic vinegar
- 1 tbsp parsley, chopped
- 1 yellow onion, chopped
- 1 celery stick, chopped
- 1 tomato, chopped
- 2 tbsp tomato paste
- 1 and ½ tsp garlic, minced
- A pinch of sea salt
- Black pepper to the taste

Directions:

1. Rub the eggplant with cooking oil and grill it for 5 minutes per side on a preheated grill.
2. Chop the grilled eggplant and transfer it to the slow cooker.
3. Add tomato, parsley, and all other ingredients to the cooker.
4. Put the cooker's lid on and set the cooking time to 4 hours on high.
5. Serve.

Nutrition:

- Calories: 110
- Fat: 1 g
- Carbs: 7 g
- Protein: 5 g

Calamari Rings Bowls

Preparation time:

15 minutes

Cooking time:

6 hours

Servings:

2 people

Ingredients:

- ½ pound calamari rings
- 1 tablespoon balsamic vinegar
- ½ tablespoon soy sauce
- 1 tablespoon sugar
- 1 cup veggie stock
- ½ teaspoon turmeric powder
- ½ teaspoon sweet paprika
- ½ cup chicken stock

Directions:

1. In your slow cooker, mix the calamari rings with the vinegar, soy sauce, and the other fixing, toss, put the lid on and cook on high for 6 hours.

2. Divide into bowls and serve right away as an appetizer.

Nutrition:

- Calories: 230
- Fat: 2 g
- Carbs: 7 g
- Protein: 5 g

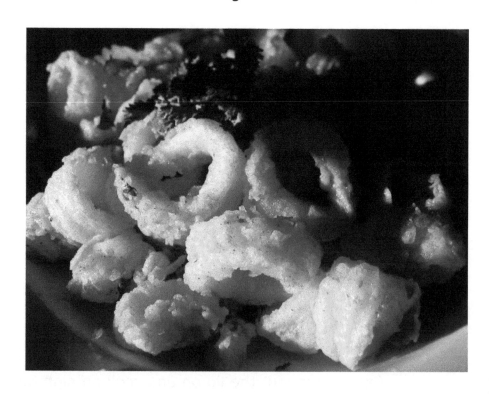